# MRCGP CSA Explanations & 2 Week Wait Referrals

## Dr Samar Bhutoria
### MBBS MRCS-DOHNS PGDipMedSci MRCGP

**Note from Author**

The book deals with topics relevant to the MRCGP CSA Examination.

The book contains simple explanations needed to approach some of the MRCGP CSA topics. I hope the book will prove useful to GP trainees, especially those who are having difficulty in passing the CSA Examination. I would encourage GP trainees to stay updated with the latest guidelines and practice the CSA stations.

Best wishes to those who are preparing for the MRCGP CSA Examination.

Dr Samar Bhutoria

# Index

## Care of people who misuse drugs and alcohol

20. Alcohol abuse

21. Opiate addiction

22. Addiction

23. Alcohol liver disease

24. Cannabis abuse

25. Diazepam

26. Methadone

## Care of people with ENT, oral, facial problems

27. Earache and otitis media

28. Sore throat

29. Tonsillectomy request

30. Labyrinthitis

31. Dizziness, Vertigo and BPPV

32. Hearing loss

33. Presbyacusis

34. Tinnitus

35. Obstructive sleep apnoea

36. Neck lump

37. Jaw pain

38. Sinusitis

39. Halitosis

40. Allergic rhinitis

41. Oral cancer

42. Hoarseness

## Care of people with eye problems

43. Red eye

44. Vision loss

45. Glaucoma

46. Uveitis

47. Cataracts

48. Chalazion

49. Blepharitis

50. Retinal detachment

## Care of people with metabolic problems

51. Chronic kidney disease

52. Diabetes

53. Pre-diabetes

54. Gestational diabetes

55. Addison's disease

56. Hypothyroid

57. Hyperthyroid

58. Goitre

59. Gynaecomastia

60. Hypercalcaemia

61. Tired all the time

62. Chronic fatigue syndrome

63. Fibromyalgia

64. Lithium

65. Weight loss

## Care of people with neurological problems

66. Headache

67. Migraine

68. Stroke

69. Ulnar nerve compression

70. Collapse and seizures

71. First Fit

72. Carpal tunnel syndrome

73. Multiple sclerosis

74. Meralgia paraesthetica

75. Parkinson's disease

76. Temporal arteritis and steroids

77. Transient ischaemic attack

78. Bitemporal hemianopia

79. Memory loss

80. Trigeminal neuralgia

81. Pins and needles

82. Tremors

## Respiratory Health

83. Chronic obstructive pulmonary disease

84. Asthma

85. Occupational asthma

86. Cough

87. Pneumonia

## Care of people with musculo-skeletal problems

88. Back pain

89. Back pain – metastasis

90. Ankylosing spondylitis

91. Meniscal injury knee

92. Achilles tendinopathy

93. Heel pain/plantar fascitis

94. Bunion

95. Osteoarthritis

96. Osteoporosis

97. Polymyalgia rheumatica

98. Rheumatoid arthritis

99. Methotrexate

100. Gout

101. Neck pain

102. Shoulder pain

124. Infections after travel – malaria

125. Lyme disease

126. Leptospirosis

127. Thread worm

128. HIV

129. Antibiotic resistance

## Haematology

130. Increased MCV - B12 / folate deficiency

131. Leukopenia

132. Thrombocytopenia

133. Pancytopenia following chemotherapy

## Two week wait referrals

134. 2 week wait Referrals

135. Bone and Soft Tissue Sarcoma

136. Brain and CNS Cancers

137. Breast Cancer

138. Childhood Cancers

139. Gastrointestinal tract cancer

140. Gynaecological cancer

141. Haematological cancer

142. Head and neck cancer

143. Lung cancer

## Index to Acronyms

AAA – Abdominal aortic aneurysm
A&E – Accident and Emergency
ABPM – Ambulatory Blood Pressure Monitoring
ACE-inh – Angiotensin Converting Enzyme Inhibitor
ACR – Albumin Creatinine Ratio
ACS – Acute Coronary Syndrome
AD – Autosomal Dominant
ADL – Activities of Daily Living
AF – Atrial Fibrillation
AIDS – Acquired Immuno Deficiency Syndrome
AMT – Abbreviated Mental Test
AR – Autosomal Recessive

BMI – Body Mass Index
BNF – British National Formulary
BP – Blood Pressure

CABG – Coronary Artery Bypass Grafting
CBT – Cognitive Behaviour Therapy
CCB – Calcium Channel Blocker
CCG – Clinical Commissioning Group
CHD – Coronary Heart Disease
CHF – Congestive Heart Failure
CKD – Chronic Kidney Disease
CNS – Central Nervous System
CO – Carbon Monoxide
COCP – Combined Oral Contraceptive Pill
COPD – Chronic Obstructive Pulmonary Disease
CSA – Clinical Skills Assessment
CT – Computerised Tomography
CVD – Cardiovascular Disease
CVS – Chorionic Villous Sampling/ Cardiovascular System
CXR – Chest Xray

DD – Differential Diagnosis
DM – Diabetes Mellitus
DUB – Dysfunctional Uterine Bleeding
DV – Domestic Violence
D&V – Diarrhoea and Vomiting
DVLA – Driver and Vehicle Licensing Agency
DVT – Deep Vein Thrombosis

ECG – Electrocardiogram
EPAU – Early Pregnancy Assessment Unit
ESR – erythrocyte sedimentation rate

FBC – Full Blood Count
FH – Family History
FSH – Follicle Stimulating Hormone
FU – Follow Up

GCA – Giant cell arteritis
GI – Gastro-intestinal
GMC – General Medical Council
GORD – Gastro-oesophageal Reflux Disease
GP – General Practice/ General Physician
GTN – Glyceryl Trinitrate
GUM – Genito Urinary Medicine

HBPM – Home Blood Pressure Monitoring
HBV – Hepatitis B Virus
HIV – Human Immunodeficiency Virus
HPV – Human Papilloma Virus
HRT – Hormone Replacement Therapy
HSV – Herpes Simplex Virus
HTN – Hypertension

ICE – Ideas, Concerns, Expectations
IMB – Inter-menstrual Bleeding
IMCA – Independent Mental Capacity Advocate
IUD – Intrauterine Device
IV – Intravenous

LARC – Long acting Reversible Contraceptive
LFT – Liver Function Test
LH – Luteinizing Hormone
LMP – Last Menstrual Period
LOC – Loss of consciousness
LPOA – Lasting Power of Attorney
LRTI – Lower Respiratory Tract Infection
LUT – Lower Urinary Tract

MDT – Multi-disciplinary Team
MI – Myocardial infarction/ischaemia
MRI – Magnetic Resonance Imaging
MS – Multiple Sclerosis

NHS – National Health Service
NRT – Nicotine Replacement Therapy
NSAID – Non Steroidal Anti Inflammatory Drugs
NSPCC – National Society for the Prevention of Cruelty to Children

OA – Osteoarthritis
OAB – Overactive Bladder
ODPS – Onset, Duration, Progression, Severity
OSA – Obstructive Sleep Apnoea
OT – Occupational Therapy
O&G – Obstetrics and Gynaecology

PA – Per Abdomen
PCB – Post Coital Bleeding
PCOS – Polycystic Ovary Syndrome

PE – Pulmonary Embolism
PID – Pelvic Inflammatory Disease
PIL – Patient Information Leaflet
PMB – Post Menopausal Bleeding
PMR – Polymyalgia Rheumatica
PNS – Peripheral Nervous System
POP – Progestogen Only Pill
PPI – Proton Pump Inhibitor
PR – Per Rectum
PS – Per Speculum
PSA – Prostate Specific Antigen
PSO – Psychological, Social, Occupational
PU – Per Urethra
PV – Per Vagina
PVD – Peripheral Vascular Disease

QOL – Quality of Life

RTA – Road Traffic Accident
RTI – Respiratory Tract Infection

SALT – Speech and Language Therapy
SE – Side effects / Socio-economic
SN – Safety Net
SOB – Shortness of Breath
SOCRATES – Site, Onset, Character, Radiation, Associations, Time, Exacerbating factors, Severity
SSRI – Selective Serotonin Reuptake Inhibitor
STI – Sexually Transmitted Infection

TB – Tuberculosis
TFT – Thyroid Function Test

U&E – Urea and Electrolytes
URTI – Upper Respiratory Tract Infection
USS – Ultrasound Scan
UTI – Urinary Tract Infection
UUT – Upper Urinary Tract

W/H2 – Weight / Height x Height
WCC – white cell count

XR - X-linked Recessive

# Cardiovascular Health

1. Stress test and B-Blocker

Stress test or Exercise Tolerance testing is a test for angina. It measures Blood Pressure and ECG ( heart activity ) while you are exercising and your heart is working harder. It lasts for about 20 minutes. BP and ECG is taken at rest followed by every minute of exercise.

Treadmill is used and the speed and incline changes to make exercise harder. The test can be stopped if you get too tired or breathless.

B-Blocker slows heart rate and should be stopped the day before the test.

2. Angina

Angina is chest pain caused by exertion due to reduced blood supply to the heart muscle due to narrowing of the blood vessels.
If angina occurs, stop exertion, rest and use GTN spray, call 999 if pain persists > 10 minutes.

You might need an angiogram. Angiogram is an Xray test which uses dyes to look at the blood vessels in the heart.

3. Heart failure

Heart failure or decreased efficiency of the heart occurs when the heart is not able to pump blood around the body as efficiently as it used to. Unfortunately, there is no cure but there are lots of medicines available to control symptoms.

4. Palpitations

Palpitations is awareness of your heartbeat. They can be caused by a variety of factors and are harmless in most cases.

5. Abdominal Aortic Aneurysm ( AAA )screening

Aorta is the main blood vessel in your body. The wall of the artery can become weak. If blood pressure increases, the wall balloons out at weak points causing aneurysm. Sometimes, this balloon ( aneurysm ) becomes bigger and bursts and can be fatal.

There is screening available for men > 65 years old. An ultrasound scan ( like pregnant women have ) is used to detect and measure AAA.
If increased size – refer to surgery
If borderline size – arrange follow up scans
If normal size – discharge

6. Atrial fibrillation

Atrial fibrillation is a common condition affecting the heart where the top two chambers or the atria beat irregularly. It is not pumping blood effectively and can cause chest pain, breathlessness and dizziness. There is a higher risk of forming a blood clot which can lead to a stroke or mini-stroke.

Calculate - CHA2DS2VASc and HASBLED scores
If CHA2DS2VASc score >/= 2 – Warfarin can be prescribed

Warfarin thins the blood and decreases risk of clots.
Disadvantages are increased risk of bleeding, interaction with food and medicines, and, regular monitoring with blood tests.

Novel Oral Anti-Coagulants are now available as alternative. They do not require regular monitoring blood tests.

7. Peripheral vascular disease ( PVD )

PVD is narrowing of the arteries due to build up of fatty deposits. This reduces the blood supply to the muscles of the limbs.
More blood supply is needed when you exercise.

8. Acute limb ischaemia

The blood supply to the leg has decreased to such an extent that there is a limb threatening emergency.

9. Varicose veins

Varicose veins are enlarged or dilated superficial veins and are very common.

10. Bradycardia

Bradycardia is slower than normal heart rate. The heart cannot pump enough blood to meet the body's needs.

# Digestive Health

### 11. Nocturnal cough and Gastric Reflux

The lower oesophageal sphincter relaxes and reflux of the gastric content occurs.
Heartburn or reflux occurs when acid moves up into food pipe and sometimes causes inflammation of the lining of the food pipe.
Acid affects the voice box causing irritation, inflammation and cough.

### 12. Coeliac disease

Coeliac disease is caused by increased sensitivity to gluten containing foods. The gut becomes inflamed and causes decreased absorption of nutrients.

### 13. Irritable bowel syndrome ( IBS )

IBS is a common condition caused by overactivity of part of the bowel. It occurs with bouts of abdominal pain, bloating and change in bowel habit.

### 14. Inflammatory bowel disease ( IBD )

IBD is long term inflammation of the the gut which relapses and remits.
There are 2 types – Ulcerative Colitis and Crohns disease.

### 15. Gallstones

Gallstones are formed when chemicals stored in the gall bladder harden to form a mass or stone. These can become trapped in a duct causing inflammation of the gall bladder.

### 16. Inguinal hernia

Inguinal hernia occurs when the contents of the abdomen protrude through a weakness in the abdominal wall.
The hernia might increase in size. Sometimes the swelling will not be able to be

reduced. This can lead to pain and this is an emergency.

## 17. Liver disease

Liver disease is common. The severity of the liver problem can vary from fatty liver ( which is reversible e.g. by stopping alcohol and lifestyle changes ) to Alcoholic Hepatitis ( inflammation of the liver ) to Liver Cirrhosis ( irreversible damage and loss of function of the liver )

## 18. Pruritus ani

Anal itching is a common condition and has many causes.

## 19. Diverticulitis

As age increases, walls of the bowel develop weak points. When pressure increases these weak areas balloon out making small pouches called diverticula.
Sometimes, these diverticula get inflamed - painful or bleeding or infected. This is called diverticulitis and may be treated with antibiotics.

## Care of people who misuse drugs and alcohol

### 20. Alcohol abuse

Harmful drinking occurs when drinking at levels which can result in damage to almost every organ in the body.

Alcohol dependence occurs when there is a strong desire to drink and there is difficulty in controlling its use despite harmful effects.

% alcohol x quantity in ml / 1000 = number of units
High risk drinking if > 50 units for men and > 35 units for women

DVLA advice – Do not drink and drive

### 21. Opiate addiction

Opiate addiction occurs with the continuous use of opiates. The brain stops producing natural painkillers with excessive use of opioids. This causes the body and the mind to become dependent on these drugs. This uncontrollable need for opioids can lead to overdose, infection, clots and even death.

### 22. Addiction

Addiction is a condition in which a person engages in an activity that can be pleasurable but the continued act becomes compulsive and interferes with ordinary life activities, health, work and relationships.

### 23. Alcohol liver disease

The liver stores energy, helps in digestion and removal of toxins and poisons and in formation of blood clots. Drinking excess alcohol can lead progressively to fatty liver, hepatitis, cirrhosis and liver failure.

### 24. Cannabis abuse

Cannabis use is illegal in the UK.

The maximum penalties -
for possession of cannabis is 5 years in prison and/or fine
for supplying or dealing in cannabis is 14 years in prison and/or fine.

## 25. Diazepam

Diazepam is addictive drug. It needs to be withdrawn gradually.
It is a crime to give, sell or possess diazepam illegally.

## 26. Methadone

Methadone is a prescribed drug used to help in heroin addiction.
It needs to be withdrawn gradually.
It is a crime to give, sell or possess methadone illegally.

# Care of people with ENT, oral, facial problems

### 27. Earache and otitis media

The ear drum is the thin skin between the outer and middle ear compartments which vibrates to pick up sounds.

During a cold, infection can occur behind the ear drum which makes the ear drum red and sore. The infection usually gets better in 2 to 3 days on its own because the immune system fights the infection.

### 28. Sore throat

Sore throat is very common and normally caused by infection such as common cold. Most are viral infections. Most resolve within a few days.

Centor criteria is used to determine the likelihood of bacterial infection and need for antibiotics for tonsillitis -
tonsillar exudate
anterior cervical lymphadenopathy
lack of cough
fever

### 29. Tonsillectomy request

There is a difference between viral sore throat and tonsillitis.

There is a criteria for consideration for tonsillectomy
Severe/disabling sore throat
>/= 7 attacks in 1 year
>/= 5 attacks each year for 2 years
>/= 3 attacks each year for 3 years
>/= 2 quinsy
sleep apnoea
increasing frequency/severity of episodes

The risk of tonsillectomy is possibility of severe bleeding

## 30. Labyrinthitis

Labyrinthitis is an inner ear infection. This affects balance.

## 31. Dizziness, Vertigo and BPPV

Dizziness and Vertigo can be due to a number of causes.

One of them is BPPV or Benign ( not serious ) Paroxysmal ( sudden ) Positional ( on movement ) Vertigo ( Dizziness )
There is an organ inside the ear which helps keep your balance. Sometimes, tiny debris can get stuck in the wrong place in this organ. This can confuse the brain and cause balance problems.

## 32. Hearing loss

Hearing loss can be due to a number of causes.
This can be a problem with the outer ear, eardrum and/or bones of the middle ear which conduct sound waves, inner ear which produces nerve signals or the brain which processes the signals.

## 33. Presbyacusis

Presbyacusis is a common condition in which there is hearing loss which develops due to increasing age.

## 34. Tinnitus

Tinnitus is the abnormal ringing or buzzing in your ear. It is common, sometimes not curable, but can be made manageable.

## 35. Obstructive sleep apnoea ( OSA )

OSA is a common condition where breathing stops for a few seconds when you are asleep. This happens when the throat muscles relax and become so floppy that they cause a temporary blockage of the airway.

## 36. Neck lump

Neck lumps can be due to a number of causes and might need investigations urgently.

Neck lumps are very commonly lymph node swellings caused by infection. They become enlarged to help us fight infection. They go back to normal in 6 weeks. If they last longer, this needs investigations as there might be a small chance of cancer.

## 37. Jaw pain

Jaw pain is common and can be caused by problems with Temporo-Mandibular Joint, ears, teeth, etc.

## 38. Sinusitis

Sinusitis is caused by inflammation of the sinuses ( air filled cavities behind cheek bones and forehead ) It is usually a viral infection and resolves in 2 to 3 weeks.

## 39. Halitosis

Halitosis or bad breath is a very common problem. It can be due to a number of causes which might need to be investigated urgently.

## 40. Allergic rhinitis

The lining of the nose gets exposed to allergens. A reaction happens and the lining of the nose gets inflamed and swollen. This can lead to nasal blockage and discharge.

## 41. Oral cancer

Abnormal lining of the inside of the mouth can be due to a number of causes and this might need to be investigated urgently.

42. Hoarseness

Hoarseness is change in voice caused by abnormal working of the vocal cords in the voice box.  This can be due to a number of causes and this might need to be investigated urgently

## Care of people with eye problems

### 43. Red eye

There are different causes of red eyes. If it is painful as well, it might require referral. The specialist will have better instruments with which they can examine your eyes such as a Slit lamp examination

### 44. Vision loss

Loss of vision can be due to various causes. These may require urgent referral to the Eye department in the hospital

### 45. Glaucoma

Glaucoma is a common condition affecting sight due to build up of pressure within the eye.

### 46. Uveitis

Uveitis is inflammation of the middle layer of the eye called the uvea or the uveal tract.

### 47. Cataracts

Cataracts is a common condition affecting the lens of the eye resulting in gradual vision loss.

### 48. Chalazion

There are glands and its ducts in the eyelid which lubricate the eyes. Obstruction of these ducts causes the glands to enlarge. Long term painless swellings are called chalazion.

## 49. Blepharitis

Blepharitis is inflammation of the margins of the eyelids


## 50. Retinal detachment

The retina is a thin layer at the back of the eye which captures light entering the eye and tells your brain what you are looking at. If this layer peels away from the back of the eye, it is called retinal detachment. This needs to be managed urgently by the specialist in the hospital.

## Care of people with metabolic problems

### 51. Chronic kidney disease ( CKD )

The kidneys filter waste from the blood and produce urine. They help to maintain Blood Pressure. With age, diabetes and high BP, the kidneys become less efficient. This efficiency is measured by a blood test called eGFR. If efficiency decreases, CKD develops if eGFR is consistently lower than normal over 3 months.

### 52. Diabetes

Diabetes is a common condition which occurs when the level of glucose in the blood becomes higher than normal. This can cause problems with eyes, feet, kidneys and heart.

It is important to adhere to treatment and know about symptoms of high and low blood sugar. It can affect driving, DVLA and insurance.

### 53. Pre-diabetes

When the level of sugar in the blood is higher than normal but not high enough to be called diabetes, it is called pre-diabetes.
If nothing is done, there is a chance that this will progress to diabetes.

### 54. Gestational diabetes

Gestational diabetes is diabetes affecting women due to pregnancy. It develops at 28 weeks and disappears when the baby is born. Screening is offered to all pregnant women with risk factors.

### 55. Addison's disease

Addison's disease is caused by destruction of the adrenal cortex which is in the adrenal gland located above the kidneys. The essential hormones regulating Blood Pressure, salt and sugar levels, immunity and stress are decreased.

## 56. Hypothyroid

Hypothyroidism is a common condition when the thyroid gland becomes underactive and does not produce enough thyroxine. Thyroxine controls the body metabolism and the body's functions slow down in hypothyroidism. Complications such as heart disease can develop and it is important to treat with thyroxine tablets.

## 57. Hyperthyroid

Hyperthyroidism occurs when the thyroid gland becomes overactive and there is raised thyroxine levels in the blood. Thyroxine controls the body metabolism which becomes faster in hyperthyroidism and causes symptoms. Complications such as heart disease can develop.

## 58. Goitre

The thyroid gland is a gland in the neck which makes a hormone called thyroxine. This keeps the body functioning at the correct rate. If the gland enlarges, it is called a goitre.

## 59. Gynaecomastia

Gynaecomastia is a common condition in which the breasts swell and become larger than normal. It can be due to age, obesity, drugs, cancer and other organ disorders.

## 60. Hypercalcaemia

Hypercalcaemia is increased calcium levels in the blood >2.65. It can affect the kidneys and the heart and can be life threatening.

## 61. Tired all the time

Tiredness is a very common problem. It can be caused by physical, psychological and lifestyle reasons. Investigations might be needed to find out the cause.

## 62. Chronic fatigue syndrome ( CFS )

Chronic fatigue Syndrome is also known as ME or Myalgic encephalomyelitis. It causes long term tiredness, sleep problems, muscle pains and headaches. There is no specific cause. Lots of help and support is available. Treatment can ease symptoms. Most people improve.

## 63. Fibromyalgia

Fibromyalgia is a long term condition causing pain all over the body. There is no cure but treatment can ease symptoms.

## 64. Lithium

Lithium is used to treat mental health disorders such as mania and bipolar disorder. It can cause side-effects and toxic levels in the blood can lead to an emergency.

## 65. Weight loss

Weight loss can be due to a number of causes which may need to be investigated urgently.

# Care of people with neurological problems

### 66. Headache

Tension headache is common and is caused by stress or physical tension. It lasts for a few hours ( range of 30 minutes to 7 days ) and is bilateral.

Cluster Headache is unilateral pain around or behind the eye, temple or forehead accompanied by eye watering and runny or congested nose. It can last from 15 to 180 minutes for few weeks to months.

Medication overuse headache can occur if medicines are taken for pain in tension headache or migraine for > 3 months. The headache occurs >15 days per month. It resolves within 2 months of stopping treatment.

### 67. Migraine

Migraine is a common type of headache caused by excited nerves which cause spasm and swelling of the blood vessels in the brain.
It can last for 1 hour to 3 days and be associated with nausea or vomiting. It may be associated with photophobia or phonophobia or both.

### 68. Stroke

A stroke is a life threatening condition caused by loss of blood supply to part of the brain ( due to bleed or clot ) leading to brain injury. Emergency hospital admission is needed.

### 69. Ulnar nerve compression

The ulnar nerve runs down the back of the upper arm. It is very close to the skin near the elbow. ( you get pins and needles when you bang your elbow )

### 70. Collapse and seizures

Collapse is caused by decreased circulation to the brain leading to loss of consciousness and vision.

Seizure is caused by a burst of abnormal electrical activity in the brain.

### 71. First Fit

Epilepsy is one of the common causes of fits and is due to abnormal electrical activity in the brain.
Patients who have a fit for the first time need to be referred to the hospital specialist urgently. They should be advised not to drive.

### 72. Carpal tunnel syndrome ( CTS )

The symptoms of CTS is caused by compression of the median nerve ( which supplies sensation to the thumb, index finger, middle finger and half of ring finger and controls some of the movements of the thumb ) as it passes through the wrist.

### 73. Multiple Sclerosis ( MS )

MS affects the nerves in the brain and spinal cord. The layer of protein which protects the nerve is damaged by the body's own immune system. This leads to intermittent disruption of the transfer of the nerve signals or messages to and from the brain and symptoms come and go.

### 74. Meralgia paraesthetica

This is caused by compression of the lateral cutaneous nerve of the thigh which supplies sensation to the surface of the skin of the thigh.

### 75. Parkinson's disease ( PD )

PD affects the brain resulting in decreased coordination of the muscle movements of the various body parts. Dopamine levels are decreased. This needs to be referred to the specialist in 2 weeks if complex problems and in 6 weeks if mild symptoms.

## 76. Temporal arteritis and steroids

Temporal arteritis is caused by inflammation of the arteries on the side of the head. It is not a common condition and can lead to blindness and stroke.
It may be associated with Polymyalgia Rheumatica (PMR), Abdominal Aortic Aneurysm (AAA) and Cardiovascular Disease (CVD).
It is an emergency condition and needs to be treated by the hospital specialist with steroids.

Advise about steroids -
Steroids may need to be taken for about 2 years. The condition can relapse after stopping steroids.
Advise to carry Steroid Card.
Advise about Side Effects – mental state change, increased Blood Pressure, weight gain, risk of infection, stomach aches, osteoporosis - advise Bone protection +/- Proton Pump Inhibitor.

## 77. Transient ischaemic attack ( TIA )

TIA or Mini-stroke occurs due to temporary lack of blood supply to part of the brain causing loss of function of brain/eyes for less than 24 hours. There is an increased risk of a stroke in the future. The risk can be decreased by initiating early treatment.

This is a warning so early treatment is needed to prevent the risk of stroke.
Calculate ABCD2 score
Age > 60 ----------------------------1

BP >/= 140/90 ---------------------1

Clinical features
Unilateral weakness ----------------2
Speech ----------------------------1
Other -----------------------------0

Duration
>/= 60 mins ------------------------2
10-59 mins-------------------------1
<10 mins --------------------------0

Diabetes ---------------------------1

High risk of stroke
ABCD2 >/= 4 ( or previous episode in last 1 week )
Refer in 24 hours

Low risk of stroke
ABCD2 </= 3
Refer to be seen in 1 week as soon as possible

Advise about driving


## 78. Bitemporal hemianopia

Bitemporal hemianopia is partial blindness where the vision is missing in the outer half of both the right and left visual fields. This may be caused by lesions in the optic nerves lying below the pituitary gland.


## 79. Memory loss

Transient Global Amnesia ( TGA ) is sudden and temporary episode of memory loss lasting less than 24 hours. There is retention of personal identity and normal cognition. There is loss of recall of recent past.


## 80. Trigeminal neuralgia

Trigeminal neuralgia (Trigeminal nerve allows you to feel your face, Neuralgia means nerve pain) is severe sudden facial pain – sharp, shooting electric shock-like pain


## 81. Pins and needles

Pins and Needles is quite common and can be due to a number of reasons which might be needed to be investigated.

## 82. Tremors

Tremor can be caused due to a number of reasons.

Essential tremor is a type of uncontrollable shake or tremble of part of the body. It is common over 40 years of age. There is no cure but treatment can help.

### 83. Chronic obstructive pulmonary disease ( COPD )

COPD is Chronic Obstructive Pulmonary Disease. As the name suggests, it is a long term condition causing irreversible obstruction of the airways. It is commonly caused by lung damage due to smoking and the most effective treatment is stopping smoking.

### 84. Asthma

Asthma affects the airways of the lungs. They become narrower and inflamed causing difficulty in breathing.

### 85. Occupational asthma

It is asthma caused by something in the workplace environment.

### 86. Cough

Cough can be due to a number of reasons. This might need to be investigated urgently.

### 87. Pneumonia

Pneumonia is a common condition. It is infection of the lung.

Use CuRB-65 ( Confusion, urea, Respiratory rate, Blood pressure, age $>/= 65$ years ) to decide management

# Care of people with musculo-skeletal problems

### 88. Back pain

Back pain is a common condition.
The most common cause is muscle sprain or a minor problem with a disc in the back bones. Serious conditions need to be ruled out.

### 89. Back pain – metastasis

Sometimes back pain can be caused by spread of cancer to the back bones from a different part of the body.

### 90. Ankylosing spondylitis ( AS )

AS is long term condition caused by inflammation of the spine and other body parts. With time, damage of the spine bones occur causing fusing of the spine called Ankylosis. It is commoner in males aged 20-30 years.

### 91. Meniscal injury knee

The menisci are rubbery pads of tissue which act as a cushion or shock absorber in the knee.
Ligaments are strong tissue in the knee which connect bones together and these get injured by a sudden pull.

### 92. Achilles tendinopathy

Achilles tendinopathy is a common condition in which the tendon which connects the calf muscles to the heel bone becomes inflamed. It can take 3 to 6 months to resolve.

### 93. Heel pain/plantar fascitis

Plantar fascitis is a common condition caused by inflammation of the plantar fascia. The plantar fascia is a strong band that stretches from the heel to the middle foot bones. It supports the foot and acts as a shock absorber. It resolves with treatment but may take 1 to 2 years to do so.

## 94. Bunion

Bunion is bony deformity at the base of the big toe.

## 95. Osteoarthritis ( OA )

OA is the wear and tear of the joint leading to inflammation causing pain and stiffness. It commonly affects knees, hips and hand joints.

## 96. Osteoporosis

Osteoporosis is a common condition when a person's bones are less dense than normal and more prone to fractures. Treatment reduces risk of fractures.

## 97. Polymyalgia rheumatica ( PMR )

PMR is a common condition causing inflammation of the large muscles in the body. This may cause pain and stiffness in the neck, shoulders, upper arms and hips.

Criteria for diagnosis -
$>/= 3$ of the following -

bilateral shoulder pain
< 2 week history
ESR > 40
morning stiffness > 1 hour
age $>/= 65$
depression +/- weight loss
bilateral tenderness in upper arm

## 98. Rheumatoid arthritis

The immune system makes antibodies against the tissues surrounding each joint leading to inflammation of the joints which causes joint damage and deformity. This is called rheumatoid arthritis and needs to be referred urgently to the specialist.

## 99. Methotrexate

Methotrexate decreases immunity thereby reducing joint inflammation and pain.

Patients need to be advised about side-effects and need for monitoring with blood tests.

Getting a sore throat while on methotrexate is serious. Methotrexate is stopped and specialist opinion is sought.

## 100. Gout

It is a common type of arthritis where uric acid crystals form inside and around joints. This causes joint inflammation and pain. Treatment is aimed at relieving symptoms and preventing future attacks.

## 101. Neck pain

There are a few causes for neck pain. Simple neck pain is when no specific cause for neck pain can be found. The symptoms can vary with physical activity and with time.

## 102. Shoulder pain

Shoulder pain can occur due to various causes.

Rotator cuff injury is damage to tissues connecting the muscle to bones.

Frozen shoulder occurs when tissues surrounding the shoulder become inflamed and stiff causing decreased movement.

OA is wear and tear of the shoulder joint.

103.    Tennis elbow

Tennis elbow is the inflammation of the tissue that connects muscle to bone on the outer part of the elbow. This is often caused by overuse of the muscle.

104.    De Quervain's tenosynovitis

De Quervain's tenosynovitis is inflammation of the tendons and its coverings on the wrist on the side of the thumb.

105.    Raynaud's disease

Raynaud's disease is a common condition when the blood vessels in your fingers/toes become narrow when you are cold causing them to change colour. The hands become red and hurt when they are warmed again. There are a few things that can be done to improve circulation.

106.    Dupuytren's contracture ( DC )

DC is a common condition when fingers bend slowly into the palm. This occurs due to thickening of the connective tissue in the palm of the hand.

# Care of people with skin problems

107.      Eczema

Eczema is a common condition of the skin which becomes dry and itchy with occasional flare-ups of inflammation. The oily barrier of the skin is reduced making it susceptible to irritants or allergens.

108.      Eczema and children

Children usually grow out of eczema.

109.      Psoriasis

Psoriasis is a common skin condition where there is increased skin production causing build up of skin forming plaques. There are occasional flare-ups.

110.      Acne

Acne is a common skin condition. There are glands in the skin that make oil to lubricate skin. Sometimes, the pores of these glands become blocked and infected causing acne. Acne generally clears with increasing age.

111.      Rosacea

Rosacea is a common skin condition affecting the face. Episodes of flushing and/or burning and tingling sensation can occur. Persistent facial redness, spots or blood vessels can also occur. There is no cure but symptoms can be kept under control with treatment.

112.      Hair loss

Hair loss is a common condition. There are many causes.

Alopecia areata mostly affects young adults. There are small patches of hair loss usually in the scalp. This resolves in a few months in most cases.

Male pattern baldness is the most common type of hair loss affecting men older than 50 years.

Telogen effluvium is a common type of hair loss with widespread thinning of the hair. This resolves in a few months in most cases.

### 113.    Itching

Itching is common and can be caused in skin conditions as well as in conditions affecting other body parts such as liver or kidneys.

### 114.    Fungal skin infection

This is a common skin condition. It can be treated with anti-fungal medication.

### 115.    Hyperhydrosis

Hyperhydrosis is excessive sweating and is a common condition.

### 116.    Rash – medication induced

Rash is a common reaction to many medicines.

### 117.    Urticaria

It is a raised itchy rash that appears on the skin. Sometimes, it can be associated with upper or lower airway obstruction or shock and is called an anaphylactic reaction.

### 118.    Allergy – peanut

Allergic reactions can be mild to severe with shortness of breath, swelling of lips or throat, collapse, etc.

Mild reactions can get worse with repeated exposure so allergen should be avoided.

Advise -
Keep calm if faced with a severe reaction.
Make sure you have help around.
Keep 2 Epipen with you at all times and use them when severe reaction occurs.
Epipen or Adrenaline opens the airways and allows ease in breathing.
Call an ambulance.
Use second epipen if no response to the first.

119.    Contact dermatitis ( CD )

CD is an inflammatory skin reaction to an irritant or allergen. It gets better in 4 to 7 days.

120.    Seborrhoeic keratosis

Seborrhoeic keratosis are very common harmless skin lesions. They appear to stick on to the skin. Their number increases with age.

121.    Melanoma

Melanoma is a type of skin cancer that can spread to other organs of the body.

# Infections

### 122.    Hepatitis C

Hepatitis C is an infection that is carried in the blood and can damage the liver. It is passed on by sharing needles, having blood transfusions with blood not checked for infections or by sexual contact.

### 123.    Shingles

Shingles is a rash caused by a virus. The chicken pox virus stays on in the nerves following an earlier infection with chicken pox. Sometimes, this sleeping chicken pox virus gets reactivated and causes a different rash called shingles. The blisters crust after 3-5 days.

### 124.    Infections after travel - malaria

Malaria is a disease spread by mosquitoes.
It can prove to be fatal if it is not treated in time.
This needs to be referred urgently to Infectious Diseases specialist

### 125.    Lyme disease

Lyme disease is a bacterial infection spread by the bite of an infected tick.

### 126.    Leptospirosis

Leptospirosis is a bacterial infection spread by handling water or soil contaminated with the urine of infected animals.

### 127.    Threadworm

Threadworms is a worm infection of the large intestine especially in children. Itching around the back passage which is worse at night is the most common symptom.

128.    Human Immunodeficiency Virus ( HIV )

HIV is a virus that attacks the immune system. Immunity decreases over a period of 10 years making the infected person more susceptible to, and, less able to, fight off infections and cancers.


129.    Antibiotic resistance

Antibiotic resistance is common with increasing use of antibiotics. The infecting organism such as a specific bacteria becomes resistant or non-responsive to the action of the antibiotic.

# Haematology

### 130.     Increased MCV - B12 / folate deficiency

The average volume of the red blood cells in body is called Mean Cell Volume. The MCV can become increased in vitamin deficiency, liver and thyroid conditions.

### 131.     Leucopenia

Leucopenia is a decrease in the disease fighting white cells in the blood. This makes the affected person vulnerable to infections.

### 132.     Thrombocytopenia

Platelets are blood cells which cause blood to clot. Thrombocytopenia is a condition in which there is a decrease in the number of platelets making the affected person prone to bruising and bleeding.

### 133.     Pancytopenia following chemotherapy

Chemotherapy kills cancer cells.
The chemicals used in chemotherapy are also toxic to the body's normal tissues such as the bone marrow which produces the blood cells. If the bone marrow is affected, there is decreased production of red and white cells and platelets. This can cause anaemia, infections and bleeding respectively.
This may be life-threatening and may need blood transfusions and antibiotics.

**Two week wait referrals**

134.      2 Week Wait Referrals

The possibility of cancer needs to be ruled out. The specialist will see you urgently in the next 2 weeks. I hope they will be able to reassure you there is no serious reason for your symptoms.

135.      Bone and Soft Tissue Sarcoma

Bone Cancer

Refer on 2 week wait -

unexplained bone swelling or pain ( needs Urgent Xray )

x-ray suggests bone sarcoma

Soft Tissue Sarcoma

Refer on 2 week wait -

unexplained lump which is increasing in size ( needs Urgent ultrasound scan )

ultrasound scan suggests soft tissue sarcoma or scan finding is uncertain

136.      Brain and CNS Cancers

Refer on 2 week wait -

loss of central neurological function ( needs MRI scan or CT scan of the Brain )

137.    Breast Cancer

Refer on 2 week wait -

Age > /= 30 years + unexplained breast lump with or without pain

Age > /= 30 years + unexplained lump in the axilla

Age > /= 50 years + changes in one nipple – nipple discharge, nipple retraction or other nipple changes

Skin changes suggestive of breast cancer

( Routine referral is needed for Age < 30 years + unexplained breast lump with or without pain )


138.    Childhood Cancers

Neuroblastoma or Wilms' Tumour -

Refer on very urgent 48 hour referral -

palpable abdominal mass

unexplained enlarged abdominal organ

unexplained visible haematuria


Retinoblastoma -

Refer on 2 week wait referral -

absent red reflex

Brain and CNS Cancer -

Refer on very urgent 48 hour referral -

new abnormal cerebellar or other central neurological function


Bone Sarcoma -

Refer on very urgent 48 hour referral -

unexplained bone swelling or pain ( needs Xray )

Xray suggests bone sarcoma


Soft Tissue Sarcoma -

Refer on very urgent 48 hour referral -

unexplained lump that is increasing in size ( needs ultrasound scan )

ultrasound scan suggests soft tissue sarcoma or ultrasound scan is uncertain


Lymphoma -

Refer on very urgent 48 hour referral -

splenomegaly

unexplained lymphadenopathy


Leukaemia -

Refer immediately to hospital if -

hepatosplenomegaly

unexplained petechiae

( Arrange urgent full blood count within 48 hours for -
generalised lymphadenopathy
pallor
unexplained fatigue / bone pain / bleeding / bruising / fever / persistent or
recurrent infection )


139.     Gastrointestinal tract cancer

Cancer of oesophagus and stomach

Refer on 2 week wait -

Age > /= 55 years + weight loss + Upper abdominal pain

Age > /= 55 years + weight loss + Reflux

Age > /= 55 years + weight loss + Dyspepsia

Dysphagia

Upper abdominal mass


( Routine Referral for UGI endoscopy is needed for -

Age > /= 55 years + Nausea or vomiting associated with either weight loss,
reflux, dyspepsia, or, upper abdominal pain

Age > /= 55 years + Raised platelet count associated with either nausea,
vomiting, weight loss, reflux, dyspepsia, or, upper abdominal pain

Age > /= 55 years + Treatment-resistant dyspepsia

Age > /= 55 years + Upper abdominal pain + low haemoglobin levels

Haematemesis )

Pancreatic cancer

Refer on 2 week wait -

Age > /= 40 years + jaundice

Age > /= 60 years + weight loss +  Abdominal pain

Age > /= 60 years + weight loss + Back pain

Age > /= 60 years + weight loss + Constipation

Age > /= 60 years + weight loss + Diarrhoea

Age > /= 60 years + weight loss + Nausea

Age > /= 60 years + weight loss + New-onset diabetes

Age > /= 60 years + weight loss + Vomiting


Cancer of gall bladder and liver

Refer on 2 week wait -

upper abdominal mass ( needs Ultrasound scan )

Colorectal cancer

Refer on 2 week wait -

Age > /= 40 years + unexplained weight loss + abdominal pain

Age > /= 50 years + unexplained rectal bleeding

Age > /= 60 years + Change in bowel habit

Age > /= 60 years + Iron-deficiency anaemia

Age < 50 years + rectal bleeding + Abdominal pain

Age < 50 years + rectal bleeding + Change in bowel habit

Age < 50 years + rectal bleeding + Iron-deficiency anaemia

Age < 50 years + rectal bleeding + Weight loss

Occult blood in faeces

Rectal or abdominal mass


140.      Gynaecological cancer

Ovarian Cancer

Refer on 2 week wait -

Ascites

Pelvic or abdominal mass (not due to uterine fibroids)

Ultrasound scan suggests ovarian cancer

( Arrange tests if any persistent symptom of -
abdominal distension or bloating
abdominal pain
change in bowel habit

fatigue

feeling full

Increased urinary frequency

Increased urinary urgency

loss of appetite

pelvic pain

unexplained weight loss

Measure serum CA125 - If serum CA125 > /= 35 IU/ml, arrange urgent ultrasound scan of the abdomen and pelvis

Refer on 2 week wait if ultrasound scan suggests ovarian cancer )

Endometrial cancer

Refer on 2 week wait -

Age > /= 55 years with post-menopausal bleeding

Age > /= 55 years + unexplained vaginal discharge + first time presenter

Age > /= 55 years + unexplained vaginal discharge + thrombocytosis

Age > /= 55 years + unexplained vaginal discharge + visible haematuria

Age > /= 55 years + visible haematuria + low haemoglobin levels

Age > /= 55 years + visible haematuria + thrombocytosis

Age > /= 55 years + visible haematuria + raised blood glucose levels

Age < 55 years with post-menopausal bleeding

Cervical cancer

Refer on 2 week wait -

Appearance of cervix suggestive of cervical cancer

( Abnormal cervical smear is referred directly to hospital by NHS Cervical Screening Programme )


Vulval cancer

Refer on 2 week wait -

unexplained vulval lump

unexplained vulval ulceration

unexplained vulval bleeding


Vaginal cancer

Refer on 2 week wait -

unexplained palpable mass in vagina

141.    Haematological cancer

## Leukaemia

Arrange urgent full blood count within 48 hours for -

generalised lymphadenopathy
hepatosplenomegaly
pallor
persistent fatigue
unexplained bleeding / bruising / fever / persistent or recurrent infection /
petechiae

## Myeloma

Arrange full blood count, calcium, plasma viscosity, erythrocyte sedimentation
rate for -

Age > /= 60 years + persistent bone pain
Age > /= 60 years + persistent back pain
Age > /= 60 years + unexplained fracture

Arrange protein electrophoresis and Bence-Jones protein urine test urgently
within 48 hours for -

Age > /= 60 years + possible myeloma + high ESR
Age > /= 60 years + possible myeloma + high plasma viscosity
Age > /= 60 years + possible myeloma + hypercalcaemia
Age > /= 60 years + possible myeloma + leukopenia

Refer on 2 week wait -

Protein electrophoresis is positive for myeloma

Bence-Jones protein urine test is positive for myeloma

Non Hodgkins lymphoma and Hodgkins lymphoma

Refer on 2 week wait -

splenomegaly

unexplained lymphadenopathy

142.      Head and neck cancer

Cancer of larynx

Refer on 2 week wait -

Age $> /= 45$ years + persistent unexplained hoarseness

Age $> /= 45$ years + unexplained lump in the neck

Oral cancer

Refer on 2 week wait -

erythroleukoplakia

lump on the lip or oral cavity

persistent unexplained lump in the neck

red or red-white patch in the oral cavity suggestive of erythroplakia

unexplained ulceration in the oral cavity $> 3$ weeks

Thyroid cancer

Refer on 2 week wait -

unexplained thyroid lump


143.    Lung cancer

Lung cancer & mesothelioma

Refer on 2 week wait -

Age > /= 40 years with unexplained haemoptysis

chest X-ray suggestive of lung cancer


Arrange Urgent 2 week wait chest X ray -

Age > /= 40 years + chest signs suggestive of cancer or pleural disease

Age > /= 40 years + finger clubbing

Age > /= 40 years + persistent or recurrent chest infection

Age > /= 40 years + supraclavicular lymphadenopathy or persistent cervical lymphadenopathy

Age > /= 40 years + thrombocytosis

Age > /= 40 years + >/= 2 of unexplained symptoms of appetite loss, chest pain, cough, fatigue, shortness of breath, weight loss

Age > /= 40 years + Asbestos exposure + >/=1 of unexplained symptoms of appetite loss, chest pain, cough, fatigue, shortness of breath, weight loss

Age > /= 40 years + Smoker/Ex-smoker + >/=1 of unexplained symptoms of appetite loss, chest pain, cough, fatigue, shortness of breath, weight loss

144.     Skin cancer

Melanoma

Refer on 2 week wait -

dermoscopy suggests melanoma

pigmented skin lesion with a weighted 7-point checklist score of >/= 3

( Major features - 2 points each
Change in size
Change in shape
Change in colour
Minor features - 1 point each
Largest diameter >/= 7 mm
Inflammation
Oozing
Change in sensation )

skin lesion suggestive of nodular melanoma

Squamous cell cancer

Refer on 2 week wait -

skin lesion suggestive of squamous cell carcinoma

Basal cell cancer

Refer on 2 week wait -

skin lesion suggestive of basal cell carcinoma if routine referral is not appropriate

145.     Urological cancer

Prostate cancer

Refer on 2 week wait -

PSA levels > the age-specific range

Prostate feels malignant on rectal examination


Arrange PSA test and do rectal examination for -
Lower urinary tract symptom
Erectile dysfunction
Visible haematuria


Bladder cancer & renal cancer

Refer on 2 week wait -

Age > /= 45 years +  Unexplained visible haematuria

Age > /= 45 years + Visible haematuria after treatment of urinary tract infection

Age > /=  60 years + unexplained non-visible haematuria + dysuria

Age > /=  60 years + unexplained non-visible haematuria + raised white cell count

( Routine referral is needed if Age > /=  60 years + recurrent or persistent unexplained urinary tract infection )

Testicular cancer

Refer on 2 week wait -

non-painful change in size or shape or texture of the testis

unexplained or persistent testicular symptoms ( needs Urgent ultrasound scan )


Penile cancer

Refer on 2 week wait -

penile mass or ulcerated lesion not linked to sexually transmitted infection

persistent penile lesion after treatment for sexually transmitted infection

unexplained or persistent symptoms affecting the penis

CPSIA information can be obtained
at www.ICGtesting.com
Printed in the USA
BVHW060521070223
657977BV00014B/578